Muscles and Energy

III

Author and Publisher
EARLE E. LIEDERMAN
305 Broadway, New York

2

MUSCLES AND ENERGY

(ORIGINAL VERSION, RESTORED)

By

EARLE LIEDERMAN

Original Publisher: Earle Liederman, 305 Broadway, New York, 1926

PUBLISHED BY O'Faolain Patriot LLC, Copyright 2011

info@PhysicalCultureBooks.com

ISBN-13: 978-1467976787

ISBN-10: 1467976784

Published in the United States of America

To Order More Copies Visit: Physical Culture Books.com

MUSCLES AND ENERGY

Tissues differ from all others. Muscles form the "flesh" or the "meat" of the body. Muscle tissue is composed of cells in the form of fibers, which vary in length and shapes. The number of these fibers that are bound together, and their length and shape, govern the size and shape of the large muscles, such as the biceps or the rectus abdominis.

There are three distinct types of muscle tissue, one being of voluntary muscles, the other two of involuntary muscles. As we cannot directly affect the involuntary muscles, we shall confine our brief discussion to the voluntary muscle tissues. These are the muscles whose fibers are arranged in masses, and have tendons at each end which attach the masses (muscles) to the covering of the bones, the periosteum.

Each muscle fiber is a long, narrow cylindrical cell. The average length of these fibers or cells is about one inch, though in the "tailor's muscle" (the sartorious), running diagonally down the front and inner surfaces of the thigh, they may be five inches in length. The thickness or diameter of the cell is from about one one-thousandth of an inch to about one four-hundredth of an inch, but the size of the cells varies appreciably in the same muscle. The largest cells are about one two-hundred and fiftieth of an inch in diameter, the smallest about one twenty-five hundredth of an inch. Each cell varies with the state of rest and activity, as will be understood soon. In men the fibers are thicker, heavier than in women; and in men whose muscles are well developed the diameter of the fibers is greater than in poorly developed men.

Each muscle fiber is composed of many little fibers or fibrillae, which are massed together in the main bulk of the muscle, but are somewhat separated at the ends. Around each fibrilla is a very thin layer of connective tissue, and around the entire fiber there is a similar layer. The fibers, too, are joined together by a layer of connective tissue, which is somewhat heavier. These layers of stronger tissue are for the purpose of holding the muscle cells and bundles together and for giving strength. They do not have the ability to contract as do muscles; but they hold the glycogen (transformed sugar) that serves as fuel for the muscles. Additional glycogen is brought to the cells by the blood, which is carried in tiny blood vessels that run lengthwise and to some extent crosswise in the muscle tissue, each fiber being in contact with minute vessels.

Around the muscle cells run a group of granular cells, somewhat like a clasp, or more like a beaded circlet. These extract from the blood and lymph certain substances and put them through definite changes so that the cells can use them for nourish¬ment. When the muscle cells contract the granules dissolve and become nutriment for the cells—not unlike giving them little wafers or pellets of condensed food.

When the muscle contracts its entire substance becomes thicker and shorter. Every cell takes part in this action and undergoes these changes, when the contraction is vigorous from strong nerve stimuli; in less vigorous contraction there may not be more than half the muscle cells that are so affected. Scientists have not yet fully determined just what change takes place to produce the contraction; but it is known that there must be some sort of an impulse travelling over the nerves to start the necessary changes. This impulse may be originated by the mind, by a blow, or by mechanical, electrical, thermal (hot or cold), or chemical irritation. In every muscle cell there is a special termination of a nerve filament, over which the impulse travels to reach the cell and make the necessary chemical change in the nucleus and granules to bring about contraction.

The musculature of your body is a complex arrangement, and something that man never can duplicate in any mechanical device. While the engines of motorcycles and automobiles, airplanes and locomotives are marvelous in their construction, designed for great speed or power or both, they cannot compare in effectiveness with the engines of your muscles. For your muscles really are engines, and work somewhat on the order of mechanical engines, but without the need for special care of each one.

You have about five hundred muscles in your body, and each muscle is composed of hundreds of thousands of tiny engines, each cell being such an engine. With each toss of the head, each movement of feeding yourself, each time you lace a shoe or take a step, throw a ball or twist your spine— with every possible movement of the thousands you are doing daily—countless thousands of these little engines are brought into action.

The food you provide for your stomach eventually supplies the charge for each tiny engine, it being carried there by the blood, instead of by the fuel-supply pipes, as in mechanical engines. Instead of spark-plugs or other sparking contraptions as in man-made engines, nerve impulses provide the "sparks" that touch off the charges in the muscle engines. The action produced is contraction of the muscle, many of the little engines of each muscle 4' exploding >' at the same time. The more that explode at the same time the greater the power—the greater the contraction—of the muscle; just as the more cylinders acting together in an automobile or airplane or other mechanical engine the greater the power and smoothness of action of such an engine.

After the discharge has taken place— after the muscle contracts—the muscle relaxes. Some of the charge of each tiny engine, imcompletely used up in the explosion, hurries back into the engine to serve as fuel again; and if the blood has been supplied with replenishing fuel, more is added, and the muscle is ready for another discharge, or contraction. The blood brings the fuel steadily to the muscle engines, in the form of oxygen and sugar and other elements. After a discharge tiny blood vessels carry off what resulted from the discharge— water and carbon dioxide, the former going to the kidneys to pass out in the urine, and the latter going to the lungs to be breathed out of the body as no longer of service, in fact, as a positive detriment to the body if it remains.

The heart keeps the blood on its circuit about the body, and blood always is about the millions of little muscle-cell engines. The more the engines have to discharge—the more the muscles contract—the more work the heart engine has to do. It pumps more blood when you work hard, less when you work easily or rest. This is because the muscle engines need more fuel when they contract often and vigorously, and the blood with its fuel is brought to them in larger quantities, or oftener. Also, the more the engines explode in contraction the more waste they throw off, and the blood must be there to carry off that waste, or the muscles become "choked." Because more oxygen is needed during exertion to cause the explosions, you have to pant or breathe faster and deeper than when at rest, so that this oxygen will be in the lungs for the blood to pick up. You must breathe faster, also, so the blood can get rid, through the lungs, of the larger amount of carbonic acid gas in the blood. And just as long as there is more of this gas than normal, you breathe faster and deeper than normal; when the balance has been restored you breathe normally again.

Now, where does the driving energy of the mus¬cles come from? In every individual there is the same number of muscles, and all have the same original structure. They all have the muscle cell or fiber as the unit; all have the bundles of fibers wrapped about with the connective tissue; all have many bundles grouped together to make the muscles as we know them; all have the tendinous attachments to the bones; all have blood flowing about and through the muscles; and all have little nerve endings in the cells to cause them to contract. Except when one is paralyzed, all are capable of moving their muscles and going from place to place, feeding themselves, nodding their heads yes or shaking them no, rolling over in bed, etc. Why is it that these movements are about the full extent of the ability of some people's muscles, while others are able to walk fifty or eighty miles a day, fight twenty three-minute rounds in the squared circle, wrestle for two or three hours with the equal of their own weight, run a marathon of over twenty- six miles in a few hours, carry half an ox, shoulder a barrel of flour, or press overhead three hundred pounds or morel What is the secret of the great strength of the athletes and strong men? Energy! Nerve force! Vitality! Virility!

Energy! But from what is energy derived? And why don't all have it?

We know that many people eat enough, so that they should be giants of strength, if quantity of food made energy. We know many who eat steaks daily who can scarcely lift their weight. We know that many exercise enough so that they should have bulging, powerful muscles, if exercise alone made these. We know that many are lying about almost all of the twenty-four hours of every day; these should have unlimited strength and energy, if rest made these qualities. You perhaps know of some who have great vitality, and yet who are not powerful, their muscles are not particularly pleasing in contour. You perhaps know many who have superb sex health, and yet they could not run a marathon nor shoulder a sack of wheat. Something else must be necessary before one can have the combination of great energy, large muscles, enormous strength. What is it?

It isn't any one factor. It is a combination of conditions that produce these desirable qualities. We shall take up but the most prominent few of them.

First of all, there must be an inherited great vitality. As I have said, we cannot add to vitality; but we can live in such a way as to allow what vitality we have to manifest itself. Most of us are born with plenty of it, if not a superabundance. The reason we do not show much of it is because we have not called upon it or have lived in such a way as to weaken it. Like energy, if we make no demands upon vitality it apparently will become less; use it, and it seems to grow. It does not: we merely awaken it and begin to tap the underlying reservoirs. There are many ways in which we can weaken the vitality.

Then, another factor for muscle strength is food. But this does not mean huge quantities of food. More food is required by the man who is developing or who is strenuously using his muscles than is needed by the man who has small muscles and who secures little or no exercise. But the needed increase in quantity of food is not nearly so great as many think necessary, and take. A good balance between all the various classes of foods is necessary, with somewhat more starch and sugars, also fats. These are the foods that provide the specific food the muscles need for their activity, and for the best results they should be as nearly natural as possible. For the one building muscle there should be a slight increase in proteins— meats, eggs, fish, fowl, nuts, cheese and milk. But as the increase in size of muscles is to a considerable extent an increase in the thickness of the individual fibers, and not so much an increase in new cells, less protein is necessary than most people use even when not building muscle.

Another factor is use of the muscles. In the human body nothing grows, after maturity, without use. The effect of stimuli upon muscle is to cause it to do the one thing it was designed to do, and that is to contract. Repeated sending of stimuli to contract causes an increased capacity for contraction: an increased *"irritability" (see footnote) which makes it possible for the muscle to contract more readily, more completely, more powerfully. At the same time, such repeated sending of impulses increases the irritability of the nerves so that they send impulses more readily, and impulses that are more positive, more powerful. Where the stimuli are more powerful and the responses more energetic, the result is bound to be an increase in work-capacity of the muscles, and an increase in size up to a certain point.

What governs this "certain point" may be several factors. One, of course, is heredity and individual limitations. A son of small people who himself is small cannot possibly develop the bulk of muscle and the gigantic strength possible to the son of large parents who himself is a mammoth. If other factors are favorable, the small man can, however, develop much larger muscles and far greater strength than where these factors are unfavorable.

NOTE: By "irritation" it should be explained that what is meant here is not a pathological condition of undue excitability, but merely the natural and wholly desirable state of susceptibility to normal impulses— the responsiveness of the tissues to physiological stimuli.

One of these other factors is type of muscle. The two extremes of types are the long, rangy type and the short, bulky type. There is considerable difference in the muscle cells in these two types. In the former the muscles are long and narrow, their individual fibers long and slender. In the latter the muscles are short and broad, the fibers short and thick; they are also more compact or capable of being developed into more compactness. It is impossible for the man of slender build of a certain height to develop the same prominence of muscles as a broader man of the same height can develop. Nor can he develop the same strength. Nevertheless, he can develop huge muscles and terrific strength if he applies himself to exercise properly and diligently. He cannot as a rule lift such weights nor develop into a wrestling giant, as can the more bulky man.

He is more suited for running, boxing, and other endurance work. In the type of work for which each is best fitted, they each can develop great endurance and energy; it is a matter of selecting the proper type of exercise work.

But I come now to a most important factor in the development of great muscles, and also of energy and strength. That factor is sex health or virility. Virility alters the nature of the muscles and their response to stimuli. The muscles of the virile man are "closer knit," more compact, their fibers more closely bunched, less stringy, their connective tissue stronger. The nuclei (what well might be called the heart of the muscle cells) are more numerous, giving greater centers for reception of stimuli. The individual muscle fibers and the entire muscle are capable of greater degrees of contraction. The granules that serve as food are present in greater abundance, thus insuring better nutrition of the cells. The blood keeps in better circulation through the muscles, thus keeping them swept more clear of waste matter, at the same time keeping more ample supplies of nutrition and fuel always convenient for them. The nerves are better nourished, have more "irritability," and send stronger impulses to the muscles.

These favorable conditions, you readily will appreciate, make it possible for the virile man to develop better muscle, larger muscle, stronger muscle—and within a shorter period of time. Men of all sizes and builds may be virile, so that it is impossible to select a particular type of muscle, in regard to external appearance, that might be called the virile type. It is more a matter of tone, alertness, compactness and yet not hardness except when contracted, and of difference between relaxed condition and contracted condition. But of two men who have exercised equally, one of superb virility and the other of deficient virility, the muscles of the former will have a far better contour, far greater strength, far more endurance.

The biceps and triceps of the virile man easily can be developed to a size that makes the well- developed forearm seem small in comparison, while the less virile man needs to exercise far more for the same results, and even then may never get his upper arm larger than his forearm. The neck of the virile man easily develops to size sixteen to nineteen, depending upon his stature, and in fact may grow to such size without exercise—as the bull's or the stallion's neck develops much more than that of the ox or the gelding— while the man low in virility can work his head off and still have a neck far from "bull neck." The thigh of the virile man develops round and tapering; and one of the characteristics frequently noted is the forward curve of its front surface instead of a straight line from the hip to the knee. The two thighs usually come in close contact, especially at their upper third, but frequently are clear to the knees.

The thigh of the non-virile man is more slender, there is less difference between the upper and lower ends, there is no forward curve to the front surface, and very frequently there is considerable separation between them, perhaps for their entire length, but especially immediately below their separation and at their lower thirds. Of course, if the sexually weak man happens to be one of the fat type—and there are many such—then his fat thighs may scrape each other and his arm may be rounded. But I am speaking of the man who is normal so far as fat is concerned.

Many youths and men become discouraged because they cannot develop muscles as large and as strong as those of others of their build, or perhaps even smaller than they. They work faithfully, expend perhaps more time than the others, take up work that should put muscle on their frames, and yet they develop painfully slowly, or fairly rapidly up to a certain point and then can go no further having stopped much below their hopes and anticipations. Many want to know why this is; they think there is something wrong with their system of exercise.

There may be need for changing their exercises to some extent; many of them exercise too much. But with many of them it will be out of the question for them to develop the same large muscles and pleasing contour, the same strength of muscle, and the same energy to expend through those muscles, until or unless they can in some way increase their virility. Some can do this, others cannot, at least sufficiently to allow them to bring about the progress in development they desire. These will have to be content with a somewhat lower degree of all these qualities of muscle that they desire. And yet there are many of these who, by persistent efforts along right lines, have produced and others are able to produce such development as to give them abundant reason to have a wholesome pride in their bodies and in the work they can do.

The effect of virility upon the muscles and upon energy is not so much that waste matter is cleared out for better action of the muscles, though doubtless there is this effect, also; but the chief effect is in providing, through the internal secretion and its effect upon every function of the body, greater stability of nerves, better fiber of muscle, more potent food for nutrition and combustion, greater resistance to fatigue, more rapid and complete recuperation.

Experiments are being conducted at this writing to get at the secret of physical endurance of athletes—to find out what it is that makes the difference between champion athletes in various sports and the ordinary or average man. These experiments take in the heart action during activity, the vital capacity, the resistance to fatigue, and what exercises will help a man to develop the highest degree of strength, energy and endurance. It is hoped by these experiments to enable physical trainers to select men scientifically as to their training possibilities and power of resistance without guesswork or with a minimum of guesswork. They hope to determine if one's superiority is due to one factor or another, or to several factors—such as superior heart action, better functioning of the respiratory system, a better ability to use the muscles and energy economically, with a minimum of wasteful effort, etc.

Since the experiments are being conducted upon an athlete who has demonstrated his superiority over many others in his line of effort (marathon running), my opinion is that not a great deal of practical value will be learned that will be of service in selecting men whose energy and athletic superiority or inferiority have not been measured in actual endeavor. If the experiments are later broadened to include all classes of men, as to physical types and musculature, condition of virility, etc., then something of considerable value may be learned and made applicable for the good of sports in general and those participating in them.

I believe there is something in men that governs their superiority in physical endeavors and that for a good while will remain undiscovered. It is the amount of energy that cannot now be measured; it is "backbone" and grit, which cannot be estimated until after being put to the test. It is the ability of the various tissues of the body to respond to un¬usual demands, and this cannot be foretold except by elaborate tests not now made. And one of the chief factors, I fully believe, is the unusual type of energy, response and chemical processes, and the greater wealth of energy reserves that are created by internal secretion of the sex glands. The quantity of this secretion cannot be measured, nor its quality estimated. The physical type of the individual in itself will not be sufficient by which to judge a man in this respect, especially since most of them would be in an undeveloped, untrained condition. The man himself will be totally unaware of a superior or inferior quality of this secretion and the energy and stamina it creates until he is put to the test.

So it is, also, with the man who is endeavoring to develop muscle bulk and specific muscle power. He may have no knowledge of a deficiency or inferiority of internal sex secretion until he fails to develop his muscles and strength by systems of exercise that should, by all the rules of exercise, bring about marked or great development; and even after failing he may not know why he failed, for there are few who can tell him. It may be that all he will be required to do to change his body so that it will respond fully to his efforts will be to conserve his sex energy. This energy may have been wasted, or at least expended by marital or extra-marital sexual indulgence, or by nocturnal losses, by spooning, by frequent mental dwelling upon sex subjects, perhaps mental masturbation, and, rarely, by physical masturbation. I say rarely, not because this is not a frequent habit, but because it usually is outgrown by the time one enters actively into sports or physical development; besides, one's energies go so wholly into the physical activities that there is much less likelihood of masturbation by the athlete or gymnast than by the one who does little exercise to use up his reserve energy.

Fatigue and exhaustion are interesting subjects. Some consider these as different degrees of the same condition—exhaustion as a later stage of fatigue. I believe there is a. difference. My opinion is that fatigue is due to the development of waste products at a more rapid rate than they can be gotten rid of, thus producing a poisoning of the nerves and muscles and a reduction of their irritability or ability to transmit stimuli and to respond to them. Whereas, exhaustion, as I see it, is due only in part to this "drugging" by fatigue poisons and wastes, being mainly due to the consumption of the stored and immediately available nourishment of fuel.

The conduction of impulses and the response to stimuli by contracting are dependent upon some sort of physical, chemical or electrical process not yet definitely understood. But they depend much upon the condition of the body's metabolism—including reception of fuel, alteration of this fuel for

actual use or for storing for later use, repair, and passing out of waste matter. And, I believe, the gonad secretion serves sufficiently as a stimulator of some of these processes and as a stabilizer of others, to have a great influence upon all of them. That is, it stimulates naturally the metabolism and the nerve and muscle conductivity and irritability for special needs, while it stabilizes these latter and the actual response and expenditure of energy and available food. Compared to an engine's "governor," it regulates the output of energy and fuel. Thus the gonad secretion has much to do with fatigue and exhaustion: the greater the quantity and the better the quality of these secretions, the greater the resistance to these phenomena; the less the quantity, the poorer the quality; the farther from normal, the greater the susceptibility, and the greater the degree the more general the fatigue and exhaustion; likewise, the slower the recovery of strength and energy.

It is impossible for one to avoid all work. Lying down is the only thing one can do and not use some of the voluntary muscles. But even while lying down the heart beats, the rib cage rises and falls in respiration, various organs are performing work necessary to the maintenance of life itself. Even rising to sit on the side of the bed, or sitting there after rising, calls into action many muscles.

The nerves during life constantly are sending impulses to the muscles, which keep them in a slight state of tension, called muscle-tonus. This state of tone varies greatly in different individuals. It is this that keeps the muscles in condition for definite response to conscious stimuli upon a fraction of a second's notice. Without it the muscles would be lifeless during rest, could be aroused but slowly, and their response by contraction would be slight compared to that which muscle-tonus makes possible.

This constant sending of impulses keeps not only the muscles in better tone and responsiveness, but the nerves also. Many things, of course, make it possible for the nerves to continue this sending of toning impulses; but I am convinced that the gonad secretion has much to do with it. Anyone who is fully virile has a better muscle tone, even if he never has exercised, than one who has little or no gonad secretion. It is this muscle tone, this partial readiness for response on demand, that makes it possible for the muscles to develop more rapidly during developmental exercises. In other words, it is the tone that indicates the ability of the muscles to develop, both in strength and size.

Hence, in order for one to develop muscles such as he desires, it is necessary for him to have gonad secretions sufficient in amount and quality to keep the nerves and muscles in proper condition for response and development, and in proper tone when at rest.

26

Here's Health

A Personally Conducted Tour Through the House We Live In—The Human Body
By EARLE LIEDERMAN

REMEMBER that old physiology book back at school? Wasn't it the dickens how we had to memorize the number of bones in the head, the hands, the feet, etc. It was enough to make a fellow dizzy, but we had to learn it just the same. That was all O.K., good stuff and very necessary, but kind of dry reading, wasn't it?

Well, if you think "HERE'S HEALTH" is anything like that, you have another think. This is a book that tells you things about your own body from head to foot, but mixes in a good story now and then and snaps things up so as to make it as interesting as your favorite novel. A well known doctor in New York read the manuscript before the book went to press. His come-back was: *"That's the finest thing I ever read. Never knew my own job was so interesting before."*

It's something you really ought to know, fellows. It will save you many a doctor's bill and will permit you to discuss a subject that every one should know, but doesn't. It has a good kick all the way through it and you will never lay it down once you start to read it.

Did you know Earle Liederman once studied to become a physician? After spending over four years at this study he suddenly gave it up, because he decided he would rather help people prevent and overcome sickness by strengthening and building up their bodies in NATURAL ways than to doctor sick people by prescribing drugs.

In the book entitled "HERE'S HEALTH" the author steps away from his usual emphasis on muscles and strength, and gives you straight-from-the-shoulder talks on physiology and hygiene.

This is one of the brightest and breeziest books of its kind ever written. Full of pep and shows another side of Earle Liederman's life.

You have always pictured Earle Liederman as a stern, serious man, who never laughs. Well, he does laugh, for he has a remarkable sense of humor, and you too will laugh at some of the comparisons and characters he portrays within these pages.

If you want to know how to take care of yourself—if you want to learn about the inside of your wonderful body, don't miss reading this gripping, intensely interesting book.

It is not the usual dull and dry and hard-to-get-interested-in treatise on physiology, but a highly interesting and entertaining book that is as easy to read as a story—and chock-full of sound common sense and helpful advice.

It covers every organ of the human anatomy—goes straight to the point about the part of each organ in the work and health of the body and shows how to keep each organ functioning at its best.

Nearly 200 pages—Price, Postpaid, $1.75

Made in the USA
Middletown, DE
10 November 2017